I0428319

Consummation Worship

A Little Book
by:

Paeti Gustav Xaviers

Copyright 2015 - All Rights Reserved

This book is dedicated to
ALL PEOPLE
with Adoration

Low and Behold, the Lord cometh quickly
and looked down upon His Holy Lands.
"Shall I Judge These?" He probably
questioned, as He became re-acclimated to
one of His most Beloved experiments.

And, after the Judgement, in accordance
with the day promised by the Holy
Scriptures, He enlightened to me in order to
correct a "bug."

HE, is the Lord, GOD
to whom
ALL PEOPLE
were warned to pray
in the name of His Sun
or
Jesus Christ
Amen.

What What You Eat!

Without intent intent of so yuckingly doing so, US PEOPLE have become a bunch of sh*t-heads, or otherwise known as can-a-bulls (cannibals). [Warning: Do NOT even think of that as a PRODUCT NAME - it's

already called "SPAM" -
so is internet Can-Spam]
You say WHAT?!

As did I upon the
revelation.

Do you realize that the
PROPER and planet
Respectful food intended
for the nourishment of

Human Kind is "PLANTS?" Any meat, or meat by-product, or dairy and dairy-product IS SUPPOSED to make you THROW UP! Telling us that IS a no-no equivalent to the "Sin of Eve in the Garden of Eden." Fish is an in-between, to nourish upon when major boosts

of protein are necessary
[Also Known As: 'For the
Purpose of "PIGGING
OUT"' - should an
INSATIABLE CRAVING
DO-DO ARISE.

So WHAT SIN DO YOU?

Me, too.

All people should begin to graduate their eating-style to "vegan," gradually. This is not an ALARM to PANIC YOU, but just that you should REALIZE that you are "Not What You Eat," - "WHAT You EAT "CONSTITUTES" HOLY WORSHIP!"

(Reference: God).

So now you say, "Oh, Sh*t!"

Well, exactly. We are all CONN-STIPULATED [Also Known as Constipated]... So, Who's laughing NOW Devil and "friends!"

God WILL NOT strike you dead as a result of this non-intentional "bug" type of thing in the program and coding of His Creation [Well, not up until the Judgement of Your Spirit as so determined by the Promised JUDGEMENT DAY], but when He

Looked Down Upon Us [note: PAST TENSE], He said "What! What! I created a bunch of cannibals?!"

But He IS sorry for the frustration, pain and sufferings us little human beans have suffered toward a "worship" of an

even GREATER sin,
"Vanity."

[Note: He also BLESSED
those who were able to
HOLD THEIR OWN and
not LOSE CONTROL of
themselves, regardless of
faith in Conventional
Religion. I.E. Not
become Gluttons.]

He blames no one: For surely He has witnessed that all religions have been confused as to what to serve at their celebration tables (during rituals) and what to eat or not eat otherwise. But LIFE is a "ritual." In fact, everything WE DO and EVERYTHING we consume; be it food, drink or tobacco, should be considerate and respectful of Him and All of Him in His Great Glory AND NOT to so gushingly feast for the pleasures of our taste buds and bellies (i.e. To BECOME 'gluttons').

So, Have a Beer (non-achoholic)! Here's to a HAPPIER and HEALTHIER beginning of the Promised Eternal Physical Human Life.

The passed is OVER... THANK GOD.

The 40 Day Fast

Modern Version:

Supplies:

Coffee Mate
Truvia
Ground Coffee
Coffee Maker
Cigarettes (full flavor 100's)
Non-Alchoholic Beer
(if desired - for taste)
Filtered Water
(not necessarily bottled)
A GOOD, soft earplug (1)

Basic Instructions:

1) Place earplug, solidly and gently in the RIGHT ear. This plug must remain in the ear throughout the fasting period, even if you take a break. The fast can be done intermittently or in one, straight 40 day period.

2) You will need to sit in a comfortable chair when consuming. A rocking chair is perfect, since you have to switch which leg you are

crossing over, depending on which consummation worship you are performing.

3) O Holy Smoke ONLY with your right hand, with the exception of when you first light the cigarette. Only verbalize "Tuh" (inhale) and "Who" or "Whom" (exhale). DO NOT put the cigarette down, such as laying it in an ashtray, while you are smoking. If grabbing a drink (cough, dry throat, or at least before and after smoke), hold

the cigarette in your left hand,
while drinking with your right
hand.

The Book of Daniel

Chapter 1: Daniel and certain Hebrews are trained in the court of Nebuchadnezzar—They eat plain food and drink no wine—God gives them knowledge and wisdom beyond all others.

3 ¶And the king spake unto Ashpenaz the master of his eunuchs, that he should bring certain of the children of Israel, and of the king's seed, and of the princes;

4) When consuming a "meal," cross your RIGHT leg over ("You shall come as *CHILDREN*"). When performing the "sacrament," cross your LEFT leg over. Hold positions until your Holy Smoke is extinguished. Be sure to dispose of cigarette butts in the ashtray at least a few times a day.

The ONLY RITUALISTIC

process, during this 40 day period, is the consummation of the sacrament. This is the first ritual which should be mastered, prior to attempting any period of prolongation. The consummation of the sacrament is relative to "O Holy Smoke," representing the consummation of the Body (it tastes like a dead body), followed by a purification, the drinking of water (at least before and after, during as necessary [cough or choke or dry mouth]).

Meal Consummation: You may consume as many meals as you are COMFORTABLE consuming during each day of the fast, without gluttonry. Food for a meal may be a "warm" meal (like the warm milk a baby might consume) or a "cold" meal (something more "solid"). Warm meals are recommended in the morning, consisting of 1-2 cups of hot coffee (cooling during smoke), with coffee mate (flavor of choice) and truvia (to taste). Coffee should be light and sweet, like a baby's milk. Cold meals may be filtered water, of course, or, as personal preference, non-alcoholic beer, or even iced coffee (still light and sweet).

Fasting periods: For the sake of calculation ease, try to go at least 24 hours with the fast, before taking a break and consuming a regular (healthy - non-glutton) meal. But don't fret. If your ear starts to hurt at all, remove the earplug, slowly and gently. This constitutes THE END of the fast, but go as long as you can. You can always START OVER. You may notice a build up of ear wax on the plug. You have thoroughly and safely cleaned your ear. Don't wash the plug. Wipe the wax off the earplug (to leave it LUBRICATED for next use [store in a non-moist covered container - such as the container the plug came in, typically] - as fasting gets easier) with a napkin or clothe. An old cloth diaper is perfect, but a hankie is also good, considering how rare it is in present times to find an old cloth diaper. DO NOT use thin paper that would leave large residue on the lubricated plug, such as tissue. A sturdy napkin is better.

Objectives:

The Sacrament - To be "hearted" by God, through Jesus Christ our Lord and Savior.

Meals - To BREATHE the physical body appendix shut, achieving total immunity to diseases and death.

www.ingramcontent.com/pod-product-compliance
Lightning Source LLC
Chambersburg PA
CBHW070933290526
45795CB00003B/1008